WALK & EAT YOURSELF THIN - HOW TO LOSE WEIGHT WHILE STILL EATING SEVERAL MEALS PER DAY (THE WALKING FOR WEIGHT LOSS & EATING PLAN TO BURN BELLY FAT FAST!)

Introduction

If you want to lose weight from your stomach, you are absolutely not alone. This book will help you to achieve your goal and explain to you how you can still eat at the same time, so no more starvation diets.

The obesity epidemic is growing, not only in America but also in many other countries as well. Being overweight is actually a serious issue as it can lead to various health problems, as well as affecting your self-confidence.

So, let's learn how to get rid of that weight. I myself love to eat, as I'm sure you do to. In the following pages you will learn that you can still eat and lose weight at the same time. There really is no need to be hungry whilst dropping pounds, so you won't have to deal with the annoyance of hunger pangs.

Personally I don't think it's worth being hungry the whole time for the sake of being thin. Food is just too enjoyable for that! Hunger is the body's natural way of telling us that we need to eat, so our instincts tell us to get food inside our stomachs as quickly as possible. So it is not a good idea to ignore our natural instincts - we must listen to our bodies and continue to eat regularly.

It is absolutely true that keeping your stomach full by eating regular meals will actually be beneficial in helping you stick to your healthy eating plan; you will end up reaching your goal a lot faster. This also means no more anguish and feeling grumpy because there will be no more hunger.

Big-name diet plans can be expensive, and everything they offer can easily be done on your own. Likewise, diet pills can be dangerous to your health because they contain lots of chemicals and lots of caffeine. The truth is you can get the same effects by being in control of your own weight loss program, and I'm going to give you lots of tips and tricks that will ensure that you succeed. Try to use your want power rather than your will power, and you will be able to achieve your goal!

The Main Reasons for Unwanted Weight Gain

Fast food is one of the main reasons for weight gain, but eating out at fast food restaurants isn't the only problem. It is also how we choose to eat when at home, and this is mainly due to how busy we all are with home and work life these days. Many people go for the easy option of eating pre-packed ready meals that contain unhealthily high amounts of fat and salt.

Our unhealthy eating is reflected in the youth of today, as 15% of all young people below the age of 19 are overweight. And this number is growing. Slow metabolism, although part of the problem, cannot be entirely to blame. There are ways to work around slow metabolism; the main problem is that we eat the wrong foods.

The truth is losing weight is actually much easier than you think, as the most sustainable method is to simply eat less and exercise more. The reason people don't stick to this is because they want super quick results, but with super quick results they may not be long lasting. It's really all about measuring the size of the portions you eat, food choice and exercise. The main key lies in understanding how your metabolism relates to your weight.

Everything You Need to Know About Metabolism

Let's learn how metabolism directly affects your weight. The truth is metabolism doesn't determine your weight alone, but weight is determined on the balance of calories burned versus calories consumed. If you overload on calories you will gain weight. Likewise, you will lose weight if you consume fewer calories. Therefore, metabolism is both the scale that regulates your energy needs and the engine that burns your calories.

Your body converts food into energy by the process that is your metabolism. The energy that your body needs to function is produced by calories combined with oxygen. Your total energy expenditure is the number of calories your body burns each day. Here is what makes up your total body energy expenditure:

Basic - Your basic functions are covered by your basic metabolic rate. The basics are growing and repairing cells, adjusting hormone levels, circulating blood, breathing and fuel for organs. This is the largest portion of energy used as it takes up two thirds to three quarters of your daily calories. This remains quite consistent for the basics needed.

Processing - A further 10% of your daily calories is used by storing, transporting, absorbing and digesting your food. Similarly to your basic needs, your body's requirement to process food stays quite consistent throughout the day.

Physical - The remainder of calories used are taken up doing physical activity such as going for a walk, playing sports or any other movement. These calories burnt can be controlled depending on how intense and frequent these activities are.

Some people might think that unwanted weight gain is the direct result of having a low metabolism, when in fact it is unlikely that they are directly related. A common reason for weight gain is an energy imbalance, where you are consuming more calories than your body burns. So, what you need to do to lose weight in this instance is to eat fewer calories and do more physical activity to burn more calories.

There are many different things that influence how many calories you require, such as the size of your body, your age and sex. You see, a larger body requires more energy and therefore more calories than a smaller body does. Muscle burns more calories and fat, so the more muscle and less fat you have the higher your metabolic rate will be. As your age increases your muscle mass decreases, and more of your weight is accounted for by fat. Also, the older you get the slower your metabolism becomes, so your calorie needs become reduced.

It is true that men have less body fat and more muscle than women do, so this is why men generally have a higher metabolic rate and burn calories faster than women do. Unfortunately, you can't actually change your own metabolism, but you can easily burn more calories by increasing the amount of exercise you do and building lean muscle.

Your energy needs are influenced by your metabolism, however it's the amount of food you consume and the amount of physical activity you partake in that actually determines the amount you weigh. All you need is the motivation to achieve your goal and the dedication to see it through, so developing the right mindset for long-term success is essential.

How To Achieve Long-Term Success

Like many things in life that we aim towards, developing the correct mindset is vital, because there is a frame of mind that must come into play when you are trying to achieve your goal of weight loss. So, we must arm ourselves with the correct information regarding our diet in order to ensure we succeed.

The right mindset will not only give you the motivation, information and commitment levels that are needed, but it will also help you overcome any temptations that try to derail you along the way. Indeed, having the right frame of mind will not only make your weight loss more exciting, easier and a lot more fun, but it will also allow you to dramatically change your lifestyle so you can live the life you want.

Our subconscious controls many of the habits we have and we are mostly unaware of them, and this is the reason why your subconscious could inadvertently destroy our good intentions. Your mindset controls your thoughts, actions and behaviour, so if we employ certain strategies we can control and steer our behaviour to get the outcome we desire. Replacing our old habits by making new associations linked with our desired outcome will help us greatly to lose weight.

You'll find that the more you try to develop the right mindset the easier it will become, and here are some helpful ways to do so:

- Clearly mark down your goals, and be honest with yourself about what weight you want to be.

- When thinking of your goals, be specific. The more specific they are the more important they will feel.

- Give yourself a deadline, because this will add an extra layer of motivation that will really push you to achieving your goal.

- Be realistic. If you aim way too high, achieving your goal may be out of your reach. So make sure you give yourself enough time to realistically get to where you want to be. To make this even easier, you could break down your goal into smaller chunks, so you could tell yourself how many pounds you want to lose over the next month. Then, when you reach this smaller goal you can just rinse and repeat until you reach your larger end goal.

- Make sure you are doing something, however small, on a daily basis. So, focus is the key here. When they are written down in clear view so you can see them every day they will be on your mind and you'll be focused on achieving them.

- Being committed is probably the most important thing, and always remember this. Never forget your reason why you want to do this in the first place, and this will help you stay committed throughout.

We can't overlook the fact that our metabolism slows down as we age, so transforming our food becomes more difficult if we don't change our eating habits and our exercise habits to make up for this. We're going to have to adjust some lifestyle habits in order to maintain our desired weight. You can absolutely achieve success in weight loss by aiming high and pushing yourself with the correct mindset. You will be able to be the person you want to be and live the life you want to live, and you can make that change by starting right this second.

Why You Don't Need To Pay For Diet Companies or Diet Pills

Although many diet companies have their plus points, they are absolutely not necessary in order to lose weight. First of all, they are rather pricey when you consider that you have to pay for the membership along with the food. While some of these diets claim to produce dramatic results, they can also be dangerous to your health. For example, the Atkins diet lets you drop weight drastically because you're consuming very low carbs. However, being able to keep the weight off with this diet becomes very difficult because you won't be able to keep the weight off once you reintroduce carbohydrates. Also, your cholesterol levels will be higher because you are eating foods that are high in fat. By not eating carbohydrates you'll find that your energy levels will be decreased, leaving you feeling tired and unmotivated because carbs are a way for your body to transform food into energy. It will also be much harder to get a decent pump during a workout, since your muscles will be much softer. A diet plan that balances out everything you need to operate your body at an optimal level is a diet plan worth doing.

Similarly, diet pills have risks associated with taking them. Because these pills do not need to be tested by the Food and Drug Administration, they can be loaded with health risks. Even if a pill is found to be hazardous to your health, the Food and Drug Administration will remove it from future sale, but this doesn't stop it from being available in the first place.

How These Pills Work

Many of these pills suppress your appetite, some claim to increase your body's ability to burn fat and reduce hunger, while others claim to help you lose weight by removing the body's fluids. They can also be addictive, as well as having the following undesired effects: sex drive disturbances, excessive sweating, blurred vision, dizziness, headaches, fever, high blood pressure, anxiety and many more.

Nothing makes you lose weight more effectively like a balanced diet and exercise. Doing it the natural way will help you grow emotionally and improve your lifestyle.

Why Balance Is Important

It's good to drink a lot of water. A lot of people don't drink as much as they need. You should really drink eight glasses of water a day, or possibly more. You see, water is a natural appetite suppressant. So if you drink a full glass of water before you consume a meal, your stomach won't need as much food to feel full. And drinking water will not make you gain weight, instead it will hydrate your body. When we don't drink enough water, and then suddenly drink a lot we start to feel bloated. So it's much better to drink it gradually throughout the day so that it's released naturally. Then you can get the added bonuses of hydration and a feeling of fullness.

The basic food groups that make up a balanced meal is what you should always aim for. As carbohydrates are the main source of energy while proteins burn fat, each meal should include a protein and a carbohydrate. Skipping meals is extremely detrimental in regards to weight loss because your metabolism needs regular meals to stay consistent. Your body thinks that it's starving if you have an erratic eating schedule, so when you do eat it stores it as fat so it can be used for energy.

Living a sedentary lifestyle and losing weight isn't possible. People who exercise lose weight more quickly than those that don't, they also live longer and generally feel better about themselves. This doesn't have to be a vigorous gym routine, but can instead be something as simple as walking for weight loss.

The simple formula to help you calculate weight loss is: intake fewer calories than what you burn on a daily basis. So, consuming 2000 calories and burning 2500 calories in one day is ideal. Cutting down loads on the amount of calories you intake so that you won't need to burn as many is not a good way to lose weight because you will be starving yourself. You'll feel weak and hungry, and you won't be eating yourself thin.

Your body needs energy, and it needs food and calories to get this energy. Thus, eating enough so you're not starving and being able to burn off what you've eaten and a bit more afterwards is key. However, if the amount of calories you burn is the same as the amount of calories that you intake, you will remain the same.

So, the simple way to lose weight and eat at the same time is to make the correct choices when it comes to food. You need to select foods that have a low calorie count but can also satisfy your hunger. Research has shown that fat contains 9 calories per gram compared to protein and carbohydrates which contain 4 calories per gram, so the more fat contained in a food the more calories. The weight of the food you eat may very well play a more significant part in satisfying hunger than fat or calories. Thus, eating high calorie or high-fat foods to feel full may not be needed but instead your stomach needs to feel weighted by a certain amount of food.

People have a tendency to eat the same weight of food on a daily basis, no matter of the amount of fat or calories that the meal contains. Your stomach has a weight that needs to be filled for you to feel full when eating. This is why consuming soup or having a glass of water before a meal reduces your appetite, and it is also why people can consume a low-fat diet and still gain weight if most of their foods are carbs and starch.

How To Eat Yourself Thin

Eating food based on the weight to calorie ratio is key to eating for weight loss. So avoid food that is full of calories and light in weight, and instead choose food that has a low calorie count but weighs a lot. The best ones to go for are vegetables and fruits, as they are heavy due to their water and fibre content plus they are low in calories.

Snack foods, although not weighing much contain a lot of calories. So they are to be avoided because you can consume a lot of them without feeling full and therefore take in a too many calories. Indeed, lightweight food with a high calorie count is arguably the worst food to eat if you are trying to lose weight, because you are not full and you have already consumed more than enough calories. A lot of people when dieting avoid eating regular size meals because they think the larger the meal the more weight they will gain, but they don't see that lightweight foods can be detrimental if high in calories.

In order to eat and lose weight at the same time, we must cut down on our carbohydrates slightly but not entirely. We need some carbs in our system so we can have the energy to partake in exercise - without any carbs in our system this would be much more difficult, and the calories would not get burnt off.

A good balance is to make sure that at least half of your calories come from fruit, vegetables, whole grains and natural starches. Whilst the remainder of your diet should be lean protein like fish and chicken. So, balance your carbs with your protein and avoid eating carbs late at night. If you are feeling lacking of energy on a certain day, you can increase your carb intake briefly to get your energy levels up again.

As far as protein is concerned, a good rule is you should consume 1 gram of protein for every pound of body weight per meal. Although that sounds very high, the protein being referred to is lean protein so there will be hardly any fat intake. It will also accelerate regular weight loss because protein speeds up your metabolism.

When considering portion sizes, it is a good idea to never eat a serving that is larger than your clenched fist. This way you won't be overdoing it and will still feel full. If you start to crave food that you love - for example biscuits, then that's fine as long as you don't overdo it. Instead of eating several, just have one. You don't have to cut out your favourite foods as long as you keep them in moderation.

To combat hunger, you should eat more meals with smaller portions instead of fewer meals with larger portions, because when you are overly hungry you tend to overeat. As far as the smaller portion sizes are concerned, women should eat five meals per day, and men should eat six. Be sure that these meals are at least two hours apart so you'll never crave food. You will soon discover the benefits, such as:

- Better absorption of the nutrients in your food.

- Better utilisation of the nutrients in your food.

- Greater muscle growth.

- Steadier blood sugar and insulin levels.

- Reduced hunger cravings.

- Less storage of body fat.

- Higher energy levels.

- Faster metabolic rate.

Foods You Should Avoid For Weight Loss

Here is a rundown of the foods that you should absolutely avoid for weight loss. These are the worst foods, and some great alternatives.

Pre-packed foods - Basically, anything in a cardboard packet you should stay away from especially if the ingredients are not pronounceable. This is because they contain a lot of chemicals which are going to be detrimental to your diet and health. Although white rice is filling, it contains a lot of starch that can slow down your weight loss, so eat brown rice instead. Another food that contains a lot of starch is pasta mixes, so instead consume whole grain pasta - it's just as tasty and much healthier.

Drinks - You should avoid sodas and anything with caffeine in it. This is because caffeine has an insulin-stimulating weight loss inhibiting effect, so stick to decaffeinated soft drinks, coffees and teas. Likewise, stay away from any beverage that contains aspartame, refined sugar or high fructose corn syrup. Because you will be drinking water as part of your weight loss plan, a slice of lemon or lime in it can add a lot of flavour.

It's okay to have one alcoholic drink with dinner, as long as you don't drink more than this because alcohol is detrimental in regards to weight loss. Even alcoholic beverages that say they have fewer calories will still make you gain weight, so moderation is essential.

Bread - White bread is also high in starch so should be steered clear of. You will still find the carbohydrates you need in whole grain bread and they are less processed. Instead of just wheat flour, make sure the bread you choose is made with whole-wheat flour, for this will make a lot of difference.

Cans and jars - Canned food and jarred food needs to be free from a lot of chemicals. Many soup mixes are very fatty, as is chicken broth, so avoid them. Luckily there are a lot of low-fat or light choices available, so go for these. There is a tremendous amount of salt and sugar in readymade tomato-based sauces, so the best option is to make your own. Don't consume canned vegetables or canned fruit, because it's already been cooked therefore has lost almost all of its good nutrients. They also have a lot of processed sugars so always stick to fresh vegetables and fresh fruit. As far as oil goes, go for extra virgin olive oil instead of any corn-based or vegetable oils.

Protein - Lean meats are the only choice because of their low-fat. Red meat isn't as good for you as white meat, but if you do eat it pick out a lean cut with the portion size no larger than your clenched fist. When it comes to fish, fresh fish is always the way to go instead of canned, and go for the lower fat types such as cod, tuna and salmon. Grilling your fish is the best way to get rid of any remaining fat, and avoid the battered or breaded variety. There is much less fat in white meats such as chicken and turkey, rather than red meat.

Milk, Cheese and Eggs - Try not to drink too much milk because it contains some facts that can lead to weight gain. But skimmed milk is the way to go over any other kind. Alas, cheese contains fat so it's not going to help your diet, but low-fat or fat-free is okay in moderation. It's fine to eat eggs, as they are high in protein but try to only use the whites and not consume the yolks. Yoghurt is desirable over cream, although fat-free sour cream is okay if used sparingly.

Fruit and veg - Luckily pretty much all fresh vegetables will do you good, and therefore you can eat as much as you want and you'll still lose weight. Steamed is the best way to cook them, followed by oven baking or grilling. As far as fruit is concerned, be wary of fruits that contain a lot of natural sugars. Peaches and oranges are two examples of these. Even though the sugar is natural, try not to consume too much because it will still be converted to fat.

When embarking on a new diet a great psychological trick is to throw out all foods that could be tempting and potentially sabotaging to your good intentions. So get rid of the processed sugar, frozen ready meals and chips.

Your New Healthy Shopping List

Making a list before you go shopping for your new diet is an excellent technique in making sure you don't get tempted and buy food that is going to be detrimental to your weight loss. Make sure you stick to your list and plan wisely and you won't slip up.

Once you decide what your new healthy meals are going to be, picking out the ingredients needed to prepare them will be easy. Just remember to include portion sizes when planning, as this is key to consistent weight loss. Because you'll be eating several smaller meals in a day, be sure to include all the meals that you'll need.

It's a great idea to eat before you go grocery shopping. Unwanted purchases tend to happen if you're hungry when food shopping, so you won't fall into this trap if you eat before you go.

Read the labels before you buy the products, so you don't get food that will be bad for your diet. Always peruse the salt, sugar and fat content, so that you're sure you're buying food that is weight friendly. Steer clear of the pre-packed meals in the frozen section, because even though they are convenient they contain many fats and additional unneeded calories.

Cooking your own meals is the way to go, and preparing from scratch is the best option. This way you will have total control over what exactly goes into your food, the amount of sugar or salt, and it'll be tastier too.

When shopping, just remember to always stay away from food that contains empty calories such as sweets, biscuits and french fries. They will give you no nutritional value, so avoid them at all costs. Follow this plan plus exercise, and you will find that you don't have to starve yourself at all in order to lose weight.

How to Optimise Losing Belly Fat by Walking

Couple the exercise of walking with the eating for weight loss techniques explained in the earlier parts of this book and you'll absolutely succeed in reaching your goal. You can dramatically change the shape of your body just by walking 10,000 steps, and this section will guide you on your way to becoming a fitter, healthier you. This simple exercise is easy on the joints and guaranteed to shed pounds and burn belly fat. You just need to stay focused on your goal and take a walk at least twice a week.

The Process of Walking to Burn Fat

Walking is a fail-proof way to alter your exercise habits. There's no gym membership, extra costs or special skills required – all you need is the open road.

Once you get into the habit of walking, you'll find that you'll still be able to eat your favourite foods. Burning off the fat will become second nature - all you need to do is put on your walking shoes and burn the fat off. It's all about routinely following an exercise program and reaping the long-term rewards.

Although 10,000 steps might at first sound like a long distance, it's actually not that far at all. It's basically just a long stroll. By walking at a steady pace you can complete this distance in about one and a half hours. It's just under five miles in distance. The speed it takes you to complete your walk can be increased dramatically if you power walk. Power walking will change your normal walks into strength training and cardio. If you engage in power walking, it will become possible to complete your 10,000 steps in one hour.

The Clever Way to Drop Pounds

Anyone can achieve their weight loss goals by walking, you just have to stick to it. It actually makes a lot more sense to walk for weight loss rather than put yourself on a strict diet because you won't have to deal with the constant food cravings. The changes you will make by walking will improve your self confidence and help you lead a happier healthier life. Rather than go through the hunger and of not eating it is much easier and more pleasurable to take a walk. When you walk for weight loss you will naturally start to develop healthier eating habits, because you are regularly exercising and you will find that you will naturally want to eat healthier too. A lot of the pressure of weight loss will be eliminated.

The True Reason Why Walking Burns Fat

When you start moving your body, you will straight away start burning fat. Your metabolism will be greatly increased due to your muscles being put into gear. In fact, studies have shown that active people even burn calories when they sleep – so ultimately you will have to do a lot less work in the long run to achieve the body shape you desire. The truth is: you can burn 150 calories in just half an hour of walking. Now, if you start power walking, this can be increased to over 400 calories in one hour. That's a figure that I think we can all be excited about. Plus, fat will continue to be burnt off even after you've finished your walk.

The Easy Way to Walk Further

Walking 10,000 steps isn't easy for everyone, straight away. Many people have to build up to it, and this is totally fine and absolutely normal. The easiest and quickest way to motivate yourself and go the distance is to use a pedometer. This convenient device straps to your leg and counts how many steps you've taken. After each walk, take a look at the amount of steps you've taken and make a serious effort to increase this by 500 steps the next time you do it. Keep this up, and you'll discover that you can walk the full 10,000 with minimal effort within a couple of weeks. This step counting will add a sense of urgency to your new exercise regime, and will also give you a great sense of satisfaction when you hit your targets. Also, your height will determine how many steps you can take in a five mile walk – so using a pedometer will give you a far more accurate number of steps, rather than just walking the miles.

Your Body Mechanics and How This Simple Exercise Sheds Pounds

In order to burn belly fat, your abdominal muscles need to be engaged. This is why walking burns belly fat — because when you do this low-impact exercise you are actually engaging your whole body including your abs. Your posture and a steady speed both help the process, because the easy effort of maintaining a straight posture will draw your core in, thus building toned muscle on your stomach. While doing this, your body will burn up fat to use as energy, and this includes your obliques because the opposite limb movements we all naturally do when walking helps to get rid of the unwanted fat at the sides of our body. Performing crunches will no longer be necessary as walking can be used to replace these tiring exercises, and can actually be far more effective, with no risk of hurting your lower back. An added bonus of this is protecting your spine. When your abdominals become stronger from walking, the opposite side of your core — the spine — will be under far less stress when lifting heavy things.

Quick Fat Burning Facts

- During your walks, longer strides will dramatically increase your body's fat burning capabilities.

- Increasing the speed of your walking will increase the toning of your abdominals.

- You are sure to shed more pounds walking fast than the same person would walking at a slower speed.

- Power walking forces you to tighten your abs and they remain tightened until you have finished.

- This increases your body's natural capabilities of burning fat because you are actually changing your body's chemical balance that in turn results in you being conditioned to burn fat.

- The whole process becomes easier and easier, resulting in less effort to maintain a toned midsection.

- After your walk while you are recovering, the process of after-burn with continue to burn those calories.

Good for the Mind As Well As the Body

Walking for exercise is also a great way to decrease our daily stresses and help to clear our mind. It also enhances our spirit and enthusiasm for life. An unusual fact is that people that suffer from stress actually retain more fat than people that have a more easy-going disposition. The reason for this is because of their increased level of cortisol. So, by exercising you will reduce your stress levels and also decrease your cortisol. With being active and healthy it's a case of the better it gets, the better it gets. Meaning you'll be able to keep the weight off whilst simultaneously maintaining a well-balanced mood.

Tips on Walking Fast

Before you embark on power walking, it's a good idea to make sure you have the correct footwear. This is important because when walking for exercise your feet need to have a good range of motion particularly in the mid part of the foot. Tracksuit bottoms or sweat pants are ideal because they reduce the friction of your thighs. The actual motion of power walking is a swing of the hips to account for the longer gate. It's because of this that joggers put far more pressure on their knees than walkers do – they bounce on their joints as they jog which is bad for the bones, whereas walkers walk with a horizontal movement, gliding forward across the ground. A good way to walk faster and therefore burn more fat is to pump your arms with each stride, as your hormones will burn far more fat when you engage your abs and buttocks at the same time.

Once You Start, It's Easy to Keep Going

Because your mood and general sense of well-being will be dramatically increased by partaking in this low-impact exercise, you'll find that instead of it feeling like a chore to carry on, you will instead find that quitting is the last thing on your mind. The new effective weight loss that comes with taking on this exercise will mean that your goal will be a lot clearer and instead of feeling like you are forcing yourself to do it, you will feel as though you are being pleasantly pulled towards it. When people take on walking for weight loss they discover that reaching their target of 10,000 steps is both exciting and satisfying. The goals are measurable, and therefore relatively easy to carry through. The increased morale and feeling of accomplishment will mean that other fitness goals will seem a lot easier to tackle. It just takes a couple of weeks to create a habit that gives you the results you've always wanted, and the results in turn will make it easy to keep up it.

Why Pre-Walk Stretching & Walking Gear Is Important

You can quite literally not only change your body shape but also change your life by walking 10,000 steps each time you walk for exercise. However, walking to burn fat is actually quite different to walking for the purpose of getting from one place to another. Your legs, abs and buttocks all have the potential to shed pounds and get in shape – and so to get the results you desire, preparing your body with stretching and getting properly dressed beforehand will bring you greater results.

Footwear

Walking is a low-impact activity on your body, but because you will be walking 10,000 steps it's a good idea to wear the correct footwear to ensure your feet are comfortable and protected. The two activities of walking and running are quite different; therefore walking shoes can alter greatly from running shoes. The reason for this is because our joints and muscles move in different ways during these activities, so a different type of support is needed. When people run they bend their knees at a larger angle than when they walk, as opposed to the horizontal fluid motion of walking. The best type of shoe for advanced walking or power walking is one with a lot of cushioning, as well as being light in weight. Feet can swell when walking 10,000 steps, so they should be roomy and flexible enough to accommodate this. When walking, we naturally touch the ground first with our heel and then roll through to push off with our toes – so it's good to get a shoe that is flexible in the middle to absorb each step.

Let the Steps Be Counted For You

Probably the best investment you'll make when taking up walking for weight loss is a pedometer, for it will do all the step counting for you. Because leg length determines the distance it will take to perform 10,000 steps, a pedometer will take all the guess work out. It will also help to push you further because it will help you determine your maximum distance and speed. The three main types of pedometer that are used are accelerometers, coiled spring devices and hairspring models. Hairspring ones need to be kept in a constant upright position so are not very reliable when it comes to walking 10,000 steps. If you go for a more high-end pedometer you'll be able to enjoy the benefits of very accurate readings, as these can be work on the wrist and will count the number of steps no matter which direction they are held. Other benefits of these devices are speed estimates, heart rate monitoring and calorie burning information. You don't have to spend a lot or get the latest model, but you should make sure it's a durable one that will help you get a decent amount of data so that you can continue to move forward and reach your goals.

How to Avoid Chaffing

Friction can be a big issue for walkers. It depends on your body shape, but shorts could cause you to chaff your inner thigh area. A good prevention for this is investing in some good workout pants – make sure the material allows for minimal thigh friction as well as being loose enough to allow a good flow of air. It's possible to buy some that actually wick sweat away so that you'll always stay dry during a walk.

Stretching

Even though the act of walking is relatively stress-free on you body, it is still possible to sustain an injury doing so, so stretching before you head out is a very good idea. Starting at the top of your body, work your way down until each major muscle group has been limbered up. This is the best order: neck, then shoulders, then mid back, then lower back, then hips, then buttocks, then thighs, then calves. Finally, stretch your ankles carefully by rolling them in small circles.

A couple of things to look out for and avoid when stretching are not to over extend the knees. Stretching them beyond a ninety degree angle is too far and will do more harm than good. Also, pulsing whilst stretching is not a good idea because a constant flow of oxygen is needed in order to loosen up your muscles. So, lean into the stretch as far as you can whilst breathing deeply and steadily. The act of pushing into the stretch after a long exhale will improve the elasticity of your muscles.

With the right mind-set, you can stay positive and proactive in your eating and exercise habits to both dramatically increase and improve your health and fitness levels.

~~~